WHY DIDN'T I LEARN ALL THIS PARENT STUFF SOONER?

A Mother-Baby Nurse's Guide

Kara Thompson

Table of Contents:

Description:

In this book, I cover all the things I wish I had known before having a baby!
I wanted to take a lot of the topics and frequently asked questions I address on my TikTok and Instagram page --as well as from my job as a nurse -- and put them all in this book to be a quick reference for parents. Bringing a baby home can seem daunting– but knowledge and preparation is key!

From my experience as a mother-baby registered nurse and mom of three, there's a lot of things I've learned over the years. I cover everything from what to bring to the hospital, baby feeding, baby sleep, what to expect bringing a newborn home, postpartum support, and more. I talk about how to advocate for yourself during what can be a difficult time in the hopes of making the transition easier!

CHAPTER 1:

What to Bring to the Hospital

I get asked this question all the time! "What do I bring to the hospital when I have a baby?!" Now this is going to vary for a lot of people, but I can safely say as a postpartum nurse, I see a lot of the items people say they are glad they brought and items they never used. Remember, you can always call the hospital ahead of time and ask them what things they carry! So first, I'm going to give my list of "definitelies," those things that you most definitely will be glad you have!

- At least 3 sets of cozy clothes (if you are getting induced or know you will have a baby in the NICU, you may want to bring even more than this). I would bring tops preferably that have buttons so you can do skin to skin or breastfeed easily. Dark colors are better if you get blood or stains on anything.
- At least 2 nursing bras if you plan to breastfeed + 2 pairs of underwear
- Depends/your own disposable briefs
- Your own toiletries (the hospital usually has everything you need, but your own are much better!). Remember hair ties and a brush (people always forget those)!
- A sound machine
- Chargers (10 feet is preferable to reach your bed).
- Slippers or flip flops (if you don't want to be barefoot in the shower).
- A belly binder (especially if you have a cesarean section).
- Snacks

- At least 3 outfits for baby (sleepers with zippers are my personal favorites as they keep baby warm and also allow easy access for medical assessments/diaper changes).
- 2 swaddles

The following are items I consider "optional," but many patients are glad they brought them!

- Your own pillow and blanket
- A Boppy/breastfeeding support pillow
- Robe
- Nightlight
- Oil diffuser (check with your hospital if they allow them as some do not).
- Your own peri bottle (some people like to bring nicer angled ones rather than the hospital kind).
- A small fan

Basically, at the end of the day, bring what YOU want and what makes YOU happy. Don't worry about bringing too much or too little, we just want you to be happy and have what you need, and if you're missing something I'm sure we'll have it at the hospital and be happy to give it to you!

CHAPTER 2:

Preparing your Home for Baby

Getting your home "baby ready" can seem like a daunting task! As far as preparing for a newborn, there are some things I highly recommend you do to be prepared. First, think about where baby is going to sleep–if you need a bassinet or pack and play for your bedroom. Think about where you are going to spend the most time in your house and plan a safe spot to set baby. If it's the living room or kitchen, consider a playmat or infant swing/chair where you can set them if need be. Remember, an infant lounger or swing is not meant for infant sleep, and infants are supposed to be supervised while in these devices. My favorite is a simple floor mat or gym as this is a firm surface that allows them to explore their movement and also practice tummy time.

Although not needed till baby gets older, go ahead and think about anchoring furniture (it's better to plan for it now than before a potential accident). Get safety locks for cabinets, ovens, etc. and electrical outlet covers. Make sure you know what your water thermostat is set to and adjust if needed.

As far as planning to make things easier on YOU when you get home, I highly suggest making what I call "baby doom boxes." Get a couple of baskets or caddies and fill them with all the feeding items, diapers, wipes, snacks for you, etc. that you think you'll need on a regular basis. I like to keep one downstairs and one upstairs so I can change a diaper wherever I am in the house without having to run around.

For your bathroom, a lot of people benefit from having a "perineum basket." I would go ahead and set this up before coming home. Fill it with briefs, pads, witch hazel spray, benzocaine spray, or whatever you imagine you'll need for bathroom care. Speaking of bathroom care, I would also get whatever laxatives or stool softeners you want to take postpartum and have them on hand. I recommend to all my patients whether a vaginal or cesarean birth to start taking them day one from the hospital. It is better to start taking them ahead of time rather than waiting until you are super uncomfortable and constipated.

A lot of moms benefit from padsicles which you can make ahead of time. Take a maxi pad and put witch hazel or aloe vera on it and freeze it. They feel amazing if you have any swelling or tearing!

I'd also consider having some freezer meals made ahead of time, or even if friends or your church can set up a meal train for you. Do not be afraid to ask people to do this for you! Most people WANT to help or bring food and this is probably one of the number one things I hear is most helpful to new parents!

CHAPTER 3:
Questions for my OB or Midwife

Choosing a provider for your delivery can be a daunting task! This can literally make or break your birth experience, and it is SO important to do your research before selecting someone. I have lots of people ask me where/how they should give birth. I think it's important to talk to your partner and also do self-reflection on what is important to YOU. What do you want your ideal birth experience to look like? Are you wanting to be unmedicated/medicated? What are your fears about birth? Are you wanting to deliver at home, a birth center, or hospital? Do you want lots of interventions/frequent monitoring during your pregnancy or a more hands-off approach?

Once you have an idea of what you want for your birth, it's time to narrow down your providers. I always highly suggest calling the labor and delivery and postpartum floor of the hospital at which you choose to deliver and ask if they can recommend a provider. Now some nurses may say they can't give you any information, but it's worth it to see if you can get their opinion (we see a very different side of providers from working with them on a regular basis). I would look into asking on mom Facebook pages, checking out the provider's background and ratings online, or asking friends to gain as much knowledge as possible.

If you think you have decided on a provider, here are some great questions you can ask them when you meet:

- What is your C section rate?

- If I am delivering at home/birth center, what situations would lead to my being transferred to a hospital? What is your transfer rate?
- Are you comfortable with my having a doula at my birth?
- What is your "on call" schedule? Who will deliver me if you are out of town?
- Are you comfortable with unmedicated births? (if that is your choice).
- What is your background and training?
- Are you comfortable with birth plans? Would you mind if I bring my plan, and we can review it together closer to my due date?

Remember, if you meet with a provider for the first time OR something comes up later and you don't feel like they are the right fit for you anymore–you can switch to another provider! Don't feel like you need to stay with one specific person or plan if things change. Be open with them if you have concerns and if you feel invalidated or aren't on the same page about the birth experience you want. You can always reassess.

CHAPTER 4:

Choosing a Pediatrician

Your pediatrician is the doctor who your child could potentially see for 18 years of their life! It's important you get along with them and that your values align. Just as I mentioned when choosing a delivery provider, evaluate what is important to you in a pediatrician. Many pediatricians will do a "meet and greet" before you have your baby where you can talk with them ahead of time to see if you like them and their practice. Be cognizant of the location of your ped office. You are going to be taking the baby for appointments potentially a lot the first few weeks and months of their life, so I would try to find an office not too far from your home. Again, thoroughly research them online as well and ask for recommendations from friends or people in your area as this can be valuable information. The following are some good questions you can ask when selecting a ped:

- Who will be rounding on us in the hospital when we have our newborn? (oftentimes it is someone else in the practice or a hospital neonatologist and not the actual pediatrician you selected).
- (If applicable)--Who will be doing my baby's circumcision in the hospital? What method does that person use?
- How often should we expect office visits with our newborn?
- (If applicable)--Are you comfortable with a delayed or adjusted vaccine schedule if that is what we choose?
- Until what age does your office see children?
- What is your policy for sick children? Do they have a special waiting area? Do you usually have availability to get them in

quickly for appointments if necessary?

CHAPTER 5:

What You Can Expect in the Hospital Postpartum

Every hospital is different when it comes to what your postpartum experience looks like. Some have combined labor, delivery, recovery, and postpartum units so you are in the same room the entire stay. Some hospitals (typically larger ones like the one where I work) split the care–so you move to a postpartum room after delivery. How their care is structured is a question you may want to ask the hospital where you plan to deliver.

It's important to find out if your hospital is "baby friendly." Typically, this means the hospital does not have a nursery you can send your baby to–so they will stay in your room the entire time. I highly encourage you to take a tour of the hospital ahead of time if possible. Many hospitals also offer virtual tours or birthing classes, and those are invaluable at getting you comfortable with your birthing environment.

Typically, right after delivery you will need fundal rubs or massages. These are often very uncomfortable, but we do them because statistically you are most at risk for hemorrhaging in the first 4 hours after delivery. The purpose is to cause your fundus (the top part of your uterus which is a muscular organ) to shrink back down and contract. This reduces the risk of bleeding. Oftentimes, the standard of practice is to do the fundal rubs on a consistent schedule (at my hospital we do them every hour for 4 hours, then every 4 hours for 24 hours, then every 12 hours until you discharge–although this can vary by hospital). I highly recommend you attempt to pee and stay on top of your scheduled medications before a fundal rub as this will help them be less painful!

It is normal for a LOT of people to come into your room that first day. You may have the doctors, nurses, lab techs, hearing screeners, lactation consultants, birth certificate and WIC personnel, or nurse managers coming in. Remember, your rest and safety should be a priority so, if appropriate, ask if you can have a "do-not-disturb" sign on your door and if care can be "clustered" to minimize interruptions.

Typically before you leave, the items we might need to check off are: discharge orders from both the OB/midwife and the pediatrician, hearing screen completed, a car seat trial, labs on both mom and baby, circumcision (if desired), all birth certificate paperwork completed, and discharge paperwork completed.

Common hold ups to discharge may include the baby needing to be on phototherapy if they have a high bilirubin, if the baby needs additional help establishing feeding, if the infant is not having appropriate pees and poops, or if mom has pain management issues.

CHAPTER 6:
What to Expect When You Go Home

When you go home, I consider the first two weeks the "survival period." This is the hardest time because you are adjusting to a totally new person in your life who basically requires 24/7 care! So please be easy on yourself–I have many tips for navigating this time.

First of all, your baby probably won't be on much of a routine or schedule yet and will possibly be going through cluster feeding (often this happens night 2). Cluster feeding is where your baby starts to get more alert and thinks, "Hey! I'm here, and I just want to eat ALL the time." Don't be surprised if your baby wants to eat every hour and just seems more fussy. Some babies don't go through this phase, but just be prepared if they do. It will pass, and I promise it usually just lasts a couple of days!

To many new parents, one of the biggest challenges is the loss of autonomy and being able to do what you want when you want to. I think this is a big contributing factor to post partum depression.

For most parents, night number two is the most surprising. This is often when baby becomes "more alert" and can seem more fussy/ hungry. So just a warning, some babies don't have an issue, but just to prepare you!

Make sure you and your partner talk ahead of time about expectations: such as giving each other time to get out of the house for a little bit and sharing responsibilities. If having family and visitors around is what will energize you, then by all means let people come and help! But also, don't be afraid to set boundaries if that's what you need! You just had a new baby–and if people TRULY care about YOU and respect you, they will understand and honor your wishes. If someone is making you feel guilty or awkward if you say "no" or set boundaries, please know it's not on you–it's on them! If you need help or are feeling overwhelmed, PLEASE reach out and talk to people about it.

Too often we feel like because we had a baby which is a blessing we can't complain or ask for help. Let me tell you, people who love and care for you WANT to help you and help with the baby! So please, let people bring food, set up a meal train, or ask them if they can clean for you.

CHAPTER 7:

Day Schedule for Baby

Some parents tell me they don't like or don't want to follow a schedule. I get that! My husband is very type B; and when we had our first, he was hesitant about following a routine. BUT, let me tell you, babies THRIVE on a routine! Once my husband saw how putting our daughter on a schedule actually made planning things easier and made life more predictable, he was sold! Even when I work in the NICU, we have babies on a schedule.

We follow the eat, play, sleep method. So baby eats, then "plays" (which for a newborn may be just a little tummy time, time on a mat, or in a swing–but just trying to keep them awake), and then sleep. I recommend changing baby's diaper before a feeding as this will help wake them up and be more alert for a feeding. As far as feeding, we typically recommend in the hospital that babies don't feed (whether breast or bottle) for longer than 30 minutes. The reason being they start to expend more energy when they go past that time. Now if you have a sick newborn or extenuating circumstances, sometimes feedings will go longer than that and that's fine–but typically we don't like to go past 30 minutes.

Please do a web search on "wake windows" because the amount of time you keep baby awake is usually based on their age (weeks and months). Essentially, there isn't a set amount of time all babies need to be awake–it varies.

You will also learn your baby's sleep cues, that's another good time to start getting them ready for nap/bed. This usually presents as fussiness, drooping eyelids, or their obviously slowing down and becoming sleepy. I always try to keep my newborns awake until their "sleep time." BUT if I notice a bunch of sleep cues, I may go ahead and put them down a little early. So pay attention to your little one and learn their signals.

Baby's sleep environment is very important. Of course, I always support safe sleep guidelines with those being: baby is sleeping on their own sleep surface (an infant safe bassinet, crib, or pack and play), on their back, and with nothing else in the crib. The room should be a cool and comfortable temperature. I highly recommend white noise (I notice babies don't sleep well with ocean waves or lullabies) loud enough where you can hear it outside the door of the room they're in. All lights off (even nightlights), door shut. I recommend swaddling newborns for all their nap and nighttime sleep (until, of course, they reach a certain age/weight or show signs of rolling when they can be transitioned to a sleep sack).

A lot of people wonder what to do if they have multiple kids and how to "stay on schedule." Babies are a lot more flexible than you realize! If you need to take baby on the go and they get a nap in the car or in your wrap, that's ok! You won't break them and it'll be ok. I typically try to recommend getting at least 1-2 naps a day in their bed at home if possible.

CHAPTER 8:

Night Time Sleep for Baby

Just like with a day-time routine, I highly recommend a nighttime or bedtime routine! This triggers your baby into knowing it's time to go to sleep. I suggest bath time first. I know a lot of people get concerned about using soap every night on a newborn, so yes, just using a little warm water is fine! Also, do I give a bath EVERY night? No! Sometimes life gets crazy, and I skip it! If I can, I at least try to take a warm, wet washcloth and give baby a quick wipe down to simulate a bath.

After bath, I typically recommend lotion if you want, cozy PJs, and then a story or song! We're just trying to use a lot of things to signal to baby, "Ok, it's time to sleep!" Then we do the last feeding for the day (of course, depending on baby's age we will or might have middle of the night feeds).

Finally, we swaddle the baby (if appropriate), lay them in bed, lights off, sound machine on, door shut. Baby may fuss or cry a bit at first, but I try to give them a couple of minutes and usually they settle on their own without me having to go back in the room. As far as middle of the night wakings, I typically give baby 3-5 minutes of crying (not just fussing) before I go in because sometimes they settle themselves. When I go back in the room, I give them a paci, say "shush," and put a hand on them. I leave the lights off and check that they are still swaddled tightly. I don't pick them up. I don't stay in the room for a prolonged time, just a minute or two. Once I leave, I consider that one wakeup.

Now if baby starts crying again in 5 minutes or in 30 minutes (any amount of time) and I repeat the process, I consider that the 2nd wake up. I will typically do this 3 times. If baby is still crying or fussing, THEN I will turn on the lights, sound machine off, unswaddle baby, change their diaper, and feed. After feeding, I return baby to bed. The process behind this is getting baby to learn to stretch feedings longer and longer and eventually be able to sleep through the night! We aren't abandoning them–we are giving them some time to try and self soothe (sometimes they just naturally wake up in the night like we do but don't necessarily need to eat and can settle themselves).

We are letting them developmentally learn to go back to sleep but comforting and feeding when they need it. As babies get older, it is healthy for them to learn to sleep and not constantly have their GI tract working all night–so that's why we want them to learn to stretch those feeds! I understand if people don't feel comfortable allowing their baby to cry for any amount of time. But this is what works for us and many of my friends and patients, so I am just sharing my experience!

CHAPTER 9:

Baby Skin

Some of the TOP questions and concerns I get as a mother-baby nurse revolve around the baby's skin. So let's talk about common baby skin conditions! I recommend Googling images of these so you won't be surprised if you notice these on your baby.

One of the most common is newborn rash. This appears almost like red, raised, pimples and can be anywhere on baby's body. It looks scary, but it really is just baby's skin reacting to being outside of your womb! Everything touching them is new and different, so they're just reacting to all the new things. We don't put anything on the rash–it usually just takes a couple of days to self-resolve!

Next is milia, they look like little white heads and are typically on baby's nose and face. Again, don't try to pop them or do anything with them–they usually will self-resolve in a few weeks!

Slate gray spots almost look like bruises but have a gray/blue color. They can be big and blotchy and most of the time present on the infant's torso. They're often most present in darker skinned babies. Again, they will typically fade in early childhood, and no treatment is required. Of course, since they look similar to bruises don't be afraid to still point them out and ask your provider to take a closer look at them if you are concerned.

Birthmarks can show up at birth or may appear within a few weeks. They can be flat or raised and are usually red in color. They can appear anywhere on the body and again, typically no treatment is required. Some may fade or disappear over time. There are many different kinds of birthmarks, and if you are concerned or notice changes with your baby's, always talk to a provider.

Stork bites are red or pink in color and are a type of birthmark that are very common. They're the result of clustered, dilated blood vessels. They're most often on the nape of baby's neck, nose, or eyelids. You might notice them get darker when your baby cries or exerts themself. Although some may be permanent, many fade when your baby becomes a toddler.

As far as lotions, shampoos, and washes–I always lean towards and love the more simple ingredients. If you can, try to get unscented products with as few ingredients as possible. Newborns can have sensitive skin, and the more gentle we can be with it the better! I know everyone loves all the cute, baby scented washes–but I've had SO many babies react poorly to it. At least for the first few months of their life, I'd go with the gentle stuff.

CHAPTER 10:

Baby Bath Time

So how do we give our little nugget a bath?! A lot of parents are scared because babies are so tiny and wiggly as newborns! I highly suggest a little baby bathtub or basin as it just makes it so much easier when they're tiny. A pro-tip I learned from the NICU is to lay a washcloth in the bottom of your bathtub and put one over baby's body too so they feel more cozy and warm while in the tub. It really helps decrease their anger at taking a bath!

Make sure to test the temperature of the water before placing baby in there. It shouldn't be HOT hot, just warm. You can always set the temperature settings on your home to make sure the water never gets too hot. The recommendation is 120 degrees or less.

We typically start from the bottom of their body and work up. I like to do their hair last. You seriously will get fast at doing it. The first time or two you might want your partner nearby to grab anything you need or to lend a hand. I promise I have RARELY met a newborn who likes bath time, so if you think you are doing something wrong because they are screaming the whole time, I promise you aren't! They often just don't like being cold and don't know what the heck is going on! So make sure your water is warm, keep the washcloth on them, and work quickly.

A reminder, we don't recommend submerging your baby in water until their umbilical cord falls off (typically this happens when they are 10-14 days old). So until then, we just recommend sponging them off (you can still put them in the infant tub if you'd like, just don't submerge that cord).

Another hot mom tip as far as the cord goes, if you notice it is close to falling off, I wouldn't put them in any cute or special outfits. Not always, but typically when the cord falls off, there may be a little bit of bleeding, and I don't want your special baby outfits ruined! It may just spot bleed for a bit, but if you notice it bleeding more than you think is normal, don't be afraid to contact your pediatrician. They may need to put a little silver nitrate on it to help close the wound.

CHAPTER 11:
Newborn's Normal Feeding and Eliminating

The first few days of life we want to pay the most attention to when baby needs to eat and how often they pee and poop. I recommend getting an app (there are tons out there) to track this, or you can get a little notebook! Those first few days can be a blur, so writing it down really helps!

We recommend a breastfed baby eat every 2-3 hours, a formula fed baby eat every 3-4 hours. At night we can let these stretches go a little longer if the pediatrician says it is ok, but make sure you check with them.

The rule of thumb we use for voids is the infant should void for as many days old they are. For example, day one of life they should have at least one void. Day 2, they should have 2 voids, and so on and so forth. Day 5 and on, they typically will have way more than 5 a day–they usually have a void every time they eat. So my main point is if your infant is a week old they should be voiding probably every 3 or 4 hours. If they only peed once all day, that would NOT be normal, and you need to let your pediatrician know.

Poops can be a little more random. Typically we like baby to go at least once every day, but sometimes this varies especially with formula fed babies. If it's been a day or two and you can tell your baby is uncomfortable, unusually fussy, their stomach is distended or firm, please let your pediatrician know. They might make suggestions for remedies you can do at home, but it's important to at least let them know if you are concerned.

Definitely let your provider know if your baby is having persistent diarrhea, vomiting, or any green/bright yellow vomit.

If your baby ever isn't feeding or voiding/pooping appropriately, I recommend checking their temperature first. If they don't feel well, then typically they're not going to eat well. Things like ear infections might not always be apparent or cause a fever, but that pressure in their ears makes it painful for them to suck. If baby is ever inconsolable and not eating I always recommend stripping them down to make sure there's nothing bothering them, check in their mouth, ears, etc.

CHAPTER 12:

Circumcision Care

Caring for your baby post circumcision can seem daunting, and many new parents express a lot of concern about it. However, it really is a lot simpler than you think! I can not stress enough to consider very carefully the decision to circumcise your infant. Please talk to your partner thoroughly, and both do your own research about it from a health, religious, and societal perspective. I have had lots of parents not really think about it until they're in the hospital and I have posed the question. They have conflicting opinions on whether or not to do it. So please make sure you both have had time to think on and discuss it.

Please ask your doctor who will be doing the circumcision and which method they will be using. The reason this is important is it determines the care you need to do after the procedure. The doctor also needs to thoroughly discuss the procedure, risks, benefits and have you sign a consent form beforehand.

You may also want to clarify with the doctor what kind of analgesic (pain relief) will be used. Some doctors use a numbing cream that sits on the penis beforehand, and some will inject lidocaine just prior to the procedure. Often sugar water will be given to the infant on a pacifier to keep them calmer during the procedure.

The procedure itself is very quick taking usually just a few minutes. Depending on where you deliver and their policy, the infant may need to stay in the nursery for a little while to have checks done for bleeding on a regular basis. Some hospitals will allow the baby to go back to your room right away, and checks can be done there.

If the Mogan or Gomco method is used, then, as far as penile care goes, whenever you change a diaper you can wipe and clean as usual. Just be gentle with the tip of the penis as it will be red and sore and probably have slight bleeding. Your hospital should give you vaseline and gauze that will go directly on top of the penis. I recommend about a quarter-size dollop of vaseline on a gauze pad. The vaseline side goes right on the penis, and then you can close up the diaper. This is done as long as the penis is red and raw in appearance until it gets crusted over (usually a few days). The purpose of the vaseline is to keep the diaper from sticking to that raw skin as it heals so it doesn't adhere and pull on the penis.

If the Plastibell method is used, then there is a small ring and string used to tie around the foreskin to cut off blood flow so that the foreskin falls off on its own. The ring should fall off after 7-10 days. If it has not, please let your pediatrician know. We do NOT use vaseline and gauze with this method like we do with the other two methods. You don't have to do anything–just leave it and watch it.

With any of the methods mentioned, please let your pediatrician know if you notice anything that doesn't seem right. Slight bleeding after the Mogan or Gomco methods is normal, but if you notice continuous bleeding or an amount that seems like too much please let your doctor know. Your baby should be voiding like normal, so if you don't notice that they do within 8 hours of their circumcision in addition to any redness of the skin spreading up their tummy, extreme fussiness, or a fever of 100.4 or greater, then please tell your pediatrician.

Something important to note is your baby may not eat well for a few feeds after their circumcision. They just usually don't feel well/are uncomfortable so don't be surprised if your typically good eater is suddenly just wanting cuddles or sleep. You still need to attempt feedings at their regular feeding times, but a change in their eating behavior is expected. If it persists for over a couple of feeding times and you notice your newborn is still not eating and they aren't peeing the appropriate amount based on their number of days of life, please tell your pediatrician.

CHAPTER 13:

Play Time

How do you "play" with a newborn? As far as schedule goes, especially when following the eat, play, sleep method, you may be wondering what you do to entertain a little newborn or infant? I remember thinking, "My baby is 1 month old, how do I "play" with her?!" You don't necessarily need to "play" with them, but the idea is trying to keep them awake and entertained by something.

I highly recommend doing tummy time, as this is a great way to build baby's neck control and let them explore the space around them. Make sure it is done supervised and on a firm surface (I like using a quilt on the floor). A lot of babies may not like tummy time and fuss or cry, and that's super normal! If we can get them to do at least 5 minutes at every play time, then we're doing great.

Putting your awake baby in a swing or bouncer is great for "play time." Take them on a little walk outside. Walk them around the house and just talk about what things are, what they do, their colors, and so on. This is great for developing baby's speech! Involve your baby in what you're doing. You don't just have to do baby activities! Babies love to see what you're doing! I've always involved my kids with cleaning and household chores–it seems silly but demonstrating normal activities for you can be great fun for them! You can play them some music, show them toys, read books, walk them around in a baby wrap, let them see themselves in the mirror–all these can be considered "play time" activities!

CHAPTER 14:

Infant Feeding + Milk and Formula Storage

A lot of parents ask me, "When can I start giving a bottle to my breastfed baby?" It really is up to you! Some parents from day one like for the non-breastfeeding partner to give a bottle of pumped milk so they can feel included. Some people need to give bottles right away because they have to go back to work. Some sources will recommend waiting until after baby is 28 days old to reduce "nipple confusion." I do typically like to recommend if you can waiting till 6-8 weeks when your supply has regulated. But really, whenever you want to introduce a bottle is up to you! I do recommend getting someone else to practice giving baby a bottle of pumped milk before you have to go back to work. Some babies may be finicky about taking a bottle for the first time if that's not what they are used to–so getting a couple of practice sessions in beforehand can be beneficial.

There are tons of rules about breast milk and formula storage such as how long they can be at room temperature, how long you can store them in the fridge or freezer, etc. These recommendations vary slightly on the source you use and research does change overtime, so I just encourage you to check out a web source like the CDC, Medela, or Kelly Mom for those guidelines. Many of these websites have a single page printout you can put on your fridge with all the info easily right there that I think is super helpful.

Be sure to check out the appropriate ways to store milk such as the right temperature to keep your fridge and freezer, and be aware how long you can keep your milk in both based on the temperature.

You can either warm your milk/formula in a designated warmer or warm it in a mug of hot water–making sure you check the temperature on the back of your hand/wrist before feeding to baby. Never warm up milk in a microwave as this can cause inconsistent heating within the bottle that could harm baby.

The amounts you feed baby are going to vary a lot by your infant's age, weight, and size. Make sure to be following your pediatrician's recommendations for amount(s) based on your baby's specific needs. I also recommend looking up a printout of suggested ounce requirements based on baby's age to keep on your fridge, so you have a baseline for how much they are supposed to eat.

CHAPTER 15:

Sleep Environment

The environment your baby sleeps in really makes a HUGE difference in their ability to get good, uninterrupted sleep. The American Academy of Pediatrics recommends baby sleep in the same room as you for the first 6 months of their life. For us personally, my kids have never slept well being in the same room with us–and the moment I put them in their own room (shared wall with us) we all slept immensely better. This was something I discussed with my pediatrician and got her approval on (our babies still had monitors on them). Please go by your pediatrician's recommendations for where your baby sleeps in the house.

I highly recommend swaddling your baby until they begin to show signs of rolling over (typically around 3 months of age). This decreases their startle reflex and prevents them from waking up to small noises or movement. Correct swaddle technique is so important! The main mistake I see new parents make is they don't swaddle tightly enough. Think about how tight and cozy your baby was in your womb! That's how they feel comfortable– so I promise you won't hurt them by wrapping them tightly! My favorite swaddles are ones made with bamboo material–they are the most stretchy and easiest for getting baby in that good, tight wrap.

A sound machine is also important in creating a good sleep environment for baby. In my work at the hospital, I see that most newborns do not do well if they are listening to lullabies or ocean waves–my favorite is white or brown noise. You ideally should have it turned up fairly loud (obviously not at a harmful level but loud enough so you can hear that it's on outside baby's room with the door shut). The American Academy of Pediatrics recommends keeping sound machines at 50 decibels or less. There are lots of apps out there that can test this for you.

When baby goes down for a nap or bedtime, we also encourage as dark an environment as possible. The release of the hormone melatonin which helps aid in sleep is triggered by darkness. This is why I don't love nightlights or a bright environment. Some babies have no issue with this–but I notice most sleep deeper and longer when in a darkened room. I don't think you need to go all out with blackout curtains, but at least some kind of shades or curtains to help with sunlight in the morning could be beneficial if you notice your little one waking early.

I also want to remind y'all of what a safe sleep environment looks like: this is baby in their OWN sleep space (bassinet, crib, or pack and play), on their back with no extra items in the crib (no blankets,pillows, toys, etc.). The only appropriate items are the swaddle around your baby and potentially a pacifier if you use one. The crib sheet should be tight fitting. The baby's mattress needs to be firm. Adult mattresses can be unsafe as they often aren't breathable, or they can be too soft in areas causing dips which put the baby at risk for rebreathing.

Do not feel guilty about doing naps in a wrap, baby carrier, or on you! That time goes by so quickly and cherish those naps they take with you, because they won't last forever. Don't feel bad if you have to do some naps "on the go." These won't "break" your baby or turn them into a bad sleeper forever.

CHAPTER 16:

Pumping and Pump Care

Two of the big questions I get asked in the hospital are, "When can I pump? How do I start building a stash of milk since I have to go back to work?" You can start pumping whenever you want to! Everyone is different. If you are feeding your infant at the breast primarily and want to start adding on pumping, I recommend you feed baby at the breast first then pump afterwards. Usually just 5-10 minutes of pumping is sufficient, but of course, you can do whatever you want.

Stimulation is the number one way to increase production (supply and demand!), so if you do pump just be aware you may overproduce (you may or may not want this to happen, just letting you know!). I usually wait to pump until after 6 weeks because your milk supply begins to self-regulate around 6-12 weeks. This is when a lot of people give up breastfeeding because they feel like there is a decline in their production–but most of the time it is your milk production just evening out to what your baby needs! If you are concerned about a drop in your production (baby has fewer wet diapers, seems fussier between feeds, not gaining weight, etc.), then please reach out to your pediatrician and a lactation consultant.

It is recommended you clean your pump parts in warm, soapy water after each use and allow the parts to air dry. If you need to sterilize pump parts and bottles, then you are supposed to do this every 24 hours (this can be done in a bottle sterilizer, pot of boiling water for 10 minutes, or microwave sterilizer bags). The latest recommendations on this are pump and bottle parts don't necessarily need to be sterilized every day unless baby was born premature, spent time in the NICU, or has a medical condition requiring this.

I recommend packing your "pump bag" a week before you return to work to make sure you have everything you need. The following are things I recommend for the bag:

- The pump
- Extra set of pump parts
- Small bottle of dish soap to clean parts
- Bottle brush
- Milk storage bags
- Breast pads
- Microwavable sterilizer bag
- Basin (optional–but you shouldn't let parts touch/soak in a work sink)
- Washcloth (to lay parts on to dry)
- A nursing bra to pump hands free

CHAPTER 17:

Breastfeeding Facts and Tips

I wanted to give you the down and dirty about everything breastfeeding–specifically stuff I wish I had known before kids and also what my first time parents usually don't know!

First of all, it is recommended that breastfed babies eat every 2-3 hours, formula fed babies every 3-4 hours. Their stomachs are the size of a marble the first day of life! So they really don't need much the first couple of days–drops can be considered a "meal."
To put this even more into perspective, 5 drops day one is considered a "meal."

Some babies (especially those born before 37 weeks or are on the smaller side) might have a harder time being able to nurse at the breast or stay alert for feedings. If you need to pump or hand express and then give via a syringe, bottle, or spoon, that is OK! Typically a lot of babies are going to be more sleepy early on, or if they have smaller mouths it can just make it harder for them to get a deep latch. I promise it gets easier as they get bigger and stronger! If you need to pump or use a nipple shield, it doesn't have to be forever. Babies get bigger and stronger and more efficient at eating with time and practice!

You want to wear a comfortable, well fitting bra (no areas compressing milk ducts as this can lead to a clogged duct).

Talk to your partner ahead of time about what supplementation options you might want to use if the need arises. Many hospitals offer donor milk which will require you to sign a consent form (we treat it almost like a medication). So think about and decide if you might want to go that route or use formula and what kind.

Most hospitals offer lactation consults even after you are discharged from the hospital (and insurance may cover it) so don't be afraid to reach out. Le Leche League is another great resource with many free services to help you. I've even called them a few times and am so grateful they're out there!

Your milk typically takes 3-5 days to "come in." Your body is designed to make small amounts of colostrum (yellowish, thicker milk high in nutrients) the first couple of days, and that can be sufficient to feed your baby! Don't be discouraged if you have to supplement! I have a lot of moms whose milk is just taking a little longer to come in, and baby needs a little help with supplementation from formula or donor milk. This doesn't mean you are ALWAYS going to have to supplement forever! Sometimes, especially if you have a coombs positive baby, a baby with high bilirubin, or a baby with sugar issues, then supplementation is needed for that extra boost to help your baby.

I don't want you to feel like a failure if you have to supplement–it is SO common those first days and even could be longer term. But it's more common than you realize and that doesn't mean there is anything wrong with you! I always encourage parents if you want to breastfeed, keep at it and ask for help and support—BUT if or when you decide it is not benefitting you physically or mentally, then do not be afraid to stop. You and your health are just as important as baby's! If you are struggling, you can't be an effective caregiver if you aren't taking care of yourself first!

If you are engorged or have edema, we always want to use cold on the breast. That is going to decrease that swelling and make it easier for milk to flow out when we feed or pump. Typically

5-10 minutes of cold before a feed is great. You can buy freezable breast gel packs, make ice diapers, or use cold cabbage leaves!. If it starts to get very hot/warm to the touch, painful, red and streaky in appearance, you feel feverish or have a temperature, it could be mastitis. It is super important to call/tell your OB promptly if you notice these signs or symptoms as they may need to put you on antibiotics.

You can take over the counter NSAIDS like Ibuprofen or even sunflower lecithin which helps emulsify milk. It is no longer recommended to aggressively massage clogged ducts, put heat on them, or use massager tools as this can worsen the inflammation. Nurse your baby on their regular schedule, it is no longer recommended to increase pumping or nursing frequency as this is just going to increase supply and potentially make the clogged duct worse. Using a Haakaa with epsom salts can also potentially worsen skin breakdown. So best tips are to feed as you normally would, ice, ibuprofen or sunflower lecithin, gentle massage, and let your provider know if your symptoms worsen or you become concerned.

CHAPTER 18:

Introducing Solids

It is recommended to introduce solids around 4-6 months of age and when your baby has good head control. I remember being so intimidated to try and do this with my first kid! I felt the need to make ALL of her purees from scratch and use all organic products. After I had my second, I definitely had to learn to let some things go and do more packaged items as well as a lot more baby-led weaning (so much easier to give him items we were eating anyway as a family rather than making him his own purees!). I suggest doing some reading up on baby-led weaning and decide if that's an option for your family, but I do think there are a lot of great benefits to it and can make food prep easier.

If you decide to make your own purees, one suggestion I have is buying ice cube trays to freeze small cubes of puree ahead of time. You don't have to give your baby much! Until they are 1 year of age, food time is just practice! Don't stress about how much they are taking–we are just trying to expose them to different tastes and textures!

Most sources recommend offering baby vegetables, meats, or more "savory" flavors first before fruits or foods that are higher in sugar. I've noticed the BIGGEST success with my kids' meal time as well as my own mental wellbeing was when I just learned to NOT CARE. By that I mean not caring if baby makes a mess, gets food all over themselves, or doesn't eat anything I made them. The calmer your attitude, the more infectious it is to your baby. Playing with and touching their food is good for them developmentally!

So even though I know it's hard (trust me, I'm a clean freak), I promise they won't throw their food or make a mess forever–let them learn to explore!

Dieticians also recommend putting smaller amounts on your baby's plate–it's less overwhelming to them, and we would rather them ask for more than waste it. I'm talking like 3 blueberries–if they gobble them up then yes, give them more! I don't make them sit there and eat if they aren't interested. Usually eating time lasts 10 minutes or less, with me not pushing them to keep sitting there and eating if they aren't interested.

CHAPTER 19:

Car Seat Safety

This is an area I get asked about often as I'm discharging new parents and their infants from the hospital. Everyone (and rightly so!) is worried if they installed their car seat safely! I highly suggest reading your car seat manual and practicing with the seat before your baby is born. This will relieve a lot of stress if you feel more comfortable getting it in and out of your car/stroller before baby is here.

Consider taking the car seat and base to a fire station or police station before birth to have a certified technician help you install it. I would call the station ahead of time to make sure they have someone on duty to help or ask when someone would be available. Even as a nurse, I still had a wonderful policeman check mine, and he was able to point out some great features and installation tips to me.

All car seats will have an expiration date or manufactured date on the bottom. If just the manufactured date is listed, check with that car seat company to see when that specific seat expires (it's usually around 5-7 years depending on the brand). Car seats are not to be used after being in an accident or if it gets wet or damaged (many car insurances or car seat companies will replace it for you). PLEASE consider carefully before accepting or buying a car seat from someone as you never know the complete history of that car seat. If a car seat has had any water exposure, etc., it could ruin its safety and integrity. That's why I caution you to be extremely careful about where you get the seat. I would never buy or accept a seat from a stranger.

All car seats are different so make sure you read and understand your manual in regard to their height and weight requirements. All car seats have different rear vs. forward facing requirements as well. A lot of people incorrectly assume age is when you make the change from rear to forward, but it is all based on height and weight.

Lastly, I want to touch on car seat trials and what those are in case your baby needs one in the hospital. It is often done with babies who fall under a certain weight cutoff, were premature, or needed to be on oxygen at any point during their stay. We put the baby in their car seat and monitor their heart rate and oxygen saturation for a designated amount of time to make sure they remain within normal parameters. If baby "fails" their trial, don't stress! Sometimes we just need to make minor adjustments to the positioning of the seat or give baby a little more time before retesting.

CHAPTER 20:

Taking Care of Yourself

I wanted to conclude this book with what I consider the most important topic of this whole book: YOU! You as the caregiver are the top priority–if you aren't taken care of, safe, and having your needs met, then you can't be an effective caregiver to your sweet baby!

Obviously you know you need sleep, good food, support, etc. to survive and thrive after having a baby, but that's easier said than done when your life now revolves around taking care of a baby 24/7.

For me, the biggest challenge that I wish someone had warned me about was my loss of autonomy. I used to be able to go wherever I wanted, whenever I wanted! And suddenly having that taken away on top of hormone changes, body changes/dysmorphia, lack of sleep, and physically healing after giving birth is a LOT. All I can promise is it gets better! I tell all my postpartum moms before discharge that the first two weeks will be the hardest, and you will feel like you're in survival mode (which you kind of are), but after that it gets a LOT better.

I think the number one way to avoid postpartum depression or anxiety is to be prepared and make a game plan ahead of time. Be talking now to your partner, family, or friends about your fears and concerns regarding your postpartum stage. Decide how you can share responsibilities with your partner. If your friends ask how they can help, go ahead and arrange a meal train. Have a friend, family, or babysitter in place you can call on if you get overwhelmed and need a break.

If you're concerned about your mental health post baby, talk to your provider ahead of time about medications or a game plan. If you know you might need an anti-anxiety medication or therapy, go ahead and get those plans in place. I, for example, had issues with mastitis with my second baby and went ahead and made sure I had phone numbers saved for lactation consultants and people I could call on if that became an issue with my third baby. Preparation is key!

It takes us 6 weeks to recover from birth, but up to 9 months to recover from pregnancy! It is a huge shift in our hormones, sleep schedule, relationships with others, not to mention our lives completely revolve around another person now! So please give yourself grace. It takes time to feel "normal" again. I tell all my patients those first couple weeks are purely survival mode! Do what feels right to YOU! If that's laying on the couch and just feeding baby and resting, do that! If it's getting a little cleaning done, do that! But don't feel like you NEED to do anything. Lean into your mom intuition because that is the best tool you have in your toolbox.

Please do not think something is wrong with you or you are unusual if you are having a hard time postpartum. Do not compare yourself to others! Some people may have resources that you don't see–family who can help, money for sitters/ housekeepers, childcare options. So if you feel like others are "doing it better than you," I promise you are doing amazing. At the end of the day if your child is fed, loved, and clean, I think you are doing an awesome job!

Made in the USA
Coppell, TX
17 January 2024

27842427R00026